NATIONAL COMPREHENSIVE CANCER CONTROL PROGRAM
Comprehensive Cancer Control in Action

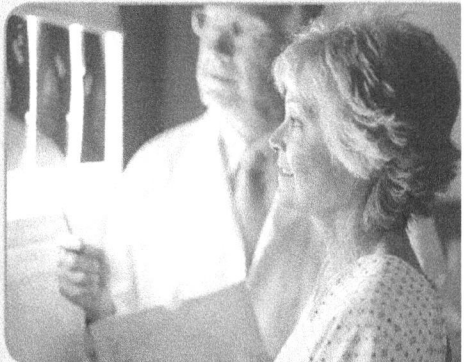

Stories OF SUCCESS

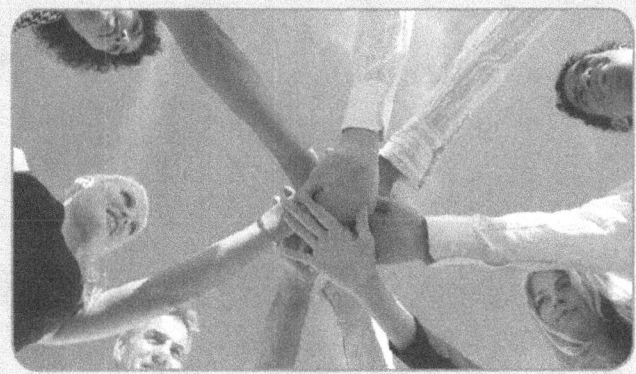

August 2012

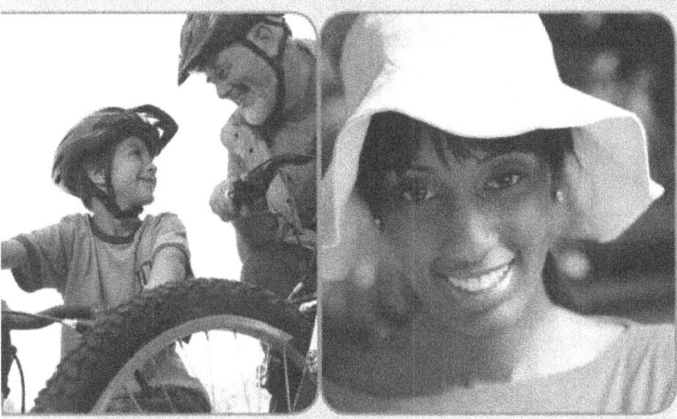

National Center for Chronic Disease Prevention and Health Promotion
Division of Cancer Prevention and Control

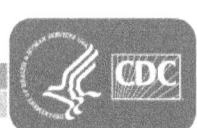

ACKNOWLEDGMENTS

We gratefully acknowledge all of the National Comprehensive Cancer Program directors, coalition coordinators, staff members, cancer survivors, community members, and other partners who submitted stories for this publication. We appreciate the time that went into crafting each submission and enjoyed reading about the many successes that are occurring across the country.

A special thanks to the program consultants of the Comprehensive Cancer Control Branch in CDC's Division of Cancer Prevention and Control (DCPC) for their assistance in collecting the success stories, to Anna Green of DCPC for providing project management support, and to Kathi Mills of DCPC for providing editorial assistance. A very special thanks to Amanda Crowell, Rick Hull, and Peggy Williams of CDC's National Center for Chronic Disease Prevention and Health Promotion for providing editorial and publishing assistance.

Suggested Citation

Centers for Disease Control and Prevention. *Stories of Success: National Comprehensive Cancer Control Program: Comprehensive Cancer Control in Action*. Atlanta: Centers for Disease Control and Prevention, National Comprehensive Cancer Control Program; 2012.

This publication is available at http://www.cdc.gov/cancer/ncccp.

A MESSAGE FROM MARCUS PLESCIA
Director, CDC's Division of Cancer Prevention and Control

Since 1999, CDC's National Comprehensive Cancer Control Program (NCCCP) has made great strides in reducing the burden of cancer in the United States. NCCCP supports states, tribes, and territories and U.S. Associated Pacific Island jurisdictions in establishing coalitions, assessing the burden of cancer, determining priorities, and developing and implementing comprehensive cancer control plans. Comprehensive cancer control programs are working in communities across the nation to promote healthy lifestyles, support recommended cancer screenings, educate people about cancer symptoms, increase access to quality cancer care, and enhance cancer survivors' quality of life.

NCCCP's success is grounded in the tremendous collaboration and valuable partnerships that reach across traditional divides to make comprehensive cancer control a reality in communities across the nation. These coalitions form an army of dedicated individuals, professionals, and cancer survivors who share expertise, resources, and ideas to tackle priorities that are too broad to confront alone. The result is a powerful nationwide network of groups collaborating to conquer cancer.

Stories of Success: Comprehensive Cancer Control in Action is a compendium of narratives that illustrate the strength of comprehensive cancer control and highlight some of the extraordinary work of NCCCP-funded programs in collaboration with their community partners. We hope they inspire readers and spark new ideas to continue NCCCP's mission.

Sincerely,

Marcus Plescia, MD, MPH
Director, Division of Cancer Prevention and Control
Centers for Disease Control and Prevention

THE HISTORY OF COMPREHENSIVE CANCER CONTROL*

In 1998, the Division of Cancer Prevention and Control at the Centers for Disease Control and Prevention established the National Comprehensive Cancer Control Program (NCCCP). This program began through the efforts of dedicated public health professionals who recognized that a more collaborative approach would be necessary to reduce the burden of cancer in the United States. They believed that coordination among those involved in the fight against cancer would have tremendous impact on prevention, early detection, treatment, quality of care, and survival.

After the "war on cancer" began in 1971, there was a gradual build up of significant cancer prevention, research, and treatment initiatives but, by the end of the 1980s, it became increasingly clear that a more comprehensive approach involving state agencies, local governments, private industry, professional organizations, voluntary organizations, the media, and others affected by cancer was needed.

In 1994, CDC, along with the American Cancer Society, the National Cancer Institute, the American College of Surgeons' Commission on Cancer, the North American Association of Central Cancer Registries, the Intercultural Cancer Council, the Chronic Disease Directors, and other public health leaders at state and national levels, began promoting a comprehensive approach that would coordinate and integrate cancer prevention and control programs across traditional funding boundaries. These organizations were later joined by C-Change (formerly the National Dialogue on Cancer) and LIVE**STRONG** (formerly the Lance Armstrong Foundation) to become the National Partnership for Comprehensive Cancer Control. A critical part of the success in developing and sustaining the new approach came from the timely and coordinated assistance from the national partners.

From 1995 to 1998, CDC held a series of meetings and workshops to gather input on the feasibility of implementing cancer control programs at the state level, and also conducted a baseline assessment of existing efforts and case studies of cancer control planning processes. Then in 1998, CDC began a pilot program that provided funding to assist five states and one tribal health board that had existing cancer control plans: Colorado, Massachusetts, Michigan, North Carolina, Texas, and the Northwest Portland Area Indian Health Board. This was the beginning of CDC's NCCCP.

Since 1998, the number of programs participating in the NCCCP has increased from six to 65. CDC awards funds to support 50 states, the District of Columbia, seven tribal governments and organizations, and seven territories and U.S. Associated Pacific Island jurisdictions in the development and implementation of their comprehensive cancer control (CCC) programs and plans.

The NCCCP, in collaboration with the national partners, supports the establishment and growth of state, tribal, territorial, and Pacific Island cancer coalitions for the development of cancer plans. These coalitions include representatives from state health departments, cancer treatment centers, local cancer organizations and taskforces, and others involved in the fight against cancer. Each coalition reviews its existing cancer data in order to develop a plan for identifying priorities and addressing cancer in that jurisdiction. The coalition then uses evidence-based strategies and activities to implement the plan. These plans are available on a Web site for CCC programs (http://cancercontrolplanet.cancer.gov).

Over the past 14 years, 64 CCC programs have begun to implement the public health strategies in their cancer plans. Cancer programs across the nation are now appreciating the impact of their accomplishments since creating their cancer plans. CDC and our national partners take pride in the achievements of the CCC programs and the effect of their activities in saving lives and building a sustainable direction for cancer prevention and control. As we continue to move forward and work with other chronic disease programs, we will continue to support the best in partnership, program evaluation, and cancer control practice, and to celebrate our success.

---

*Excerpted from Major A, Stewart SL. Celebrating 10 years of the National Comprehensive Cancer Control Program, 1998 to 2008. *Prev Chronic Dis* 2009;6(4):A133. Available at http://www.cdc.gov/pcd/issues/2009/oct/09_0072.htm.

THE POWER OF PARTNERSHIP: THE ESSENCE OF THE NATIONAL COMPREHENSIVE CANCER CONTROL PROGRAM

Collaborating to conquer cancer is the underlying philosophy, infrastructure, and focus that directs and supports CDC's National Comprehensive Cancer Control Program (NCCCP). Partners in comprehensive cancer control identify the cancer burden, plan effective interventions, conduct activities, and assess the impact of their efforts in achieving their cancer control objectives.

The stories in this compendium are examples of how states, tribes, territories, and U.S. Associated Pacific Island jurisdictions can work with partners to implement programs that contribute to their cancer goals. The voices of 17 comprehensive cancer control programs describe accomplishments along the road to reaching their ultimate goal: conquering cancer.

The Many Uses of Success Stories

Success stories are a way to share the accomplishments of the NCCCP and your state or tribal program. Success stories also provide an opportunity for those working in comprehensive cancer control to learn from others and adapt strategies to fit their program goals.

We asked NCCCP grantees and their partners to share how they planned to use their stories. Their responses included:

- Local conferences.
- Community reports.
- Grantee's meetings.
- Annual report to CDC.
- Peer-to-peer sharing.
- Stakeholder webinar.
- Community outreach.
- Creating statewide end-of-life education.
- Online and print newsletters and other publications.
- Annual report.
- Stakeholder meetings and staff trainings.

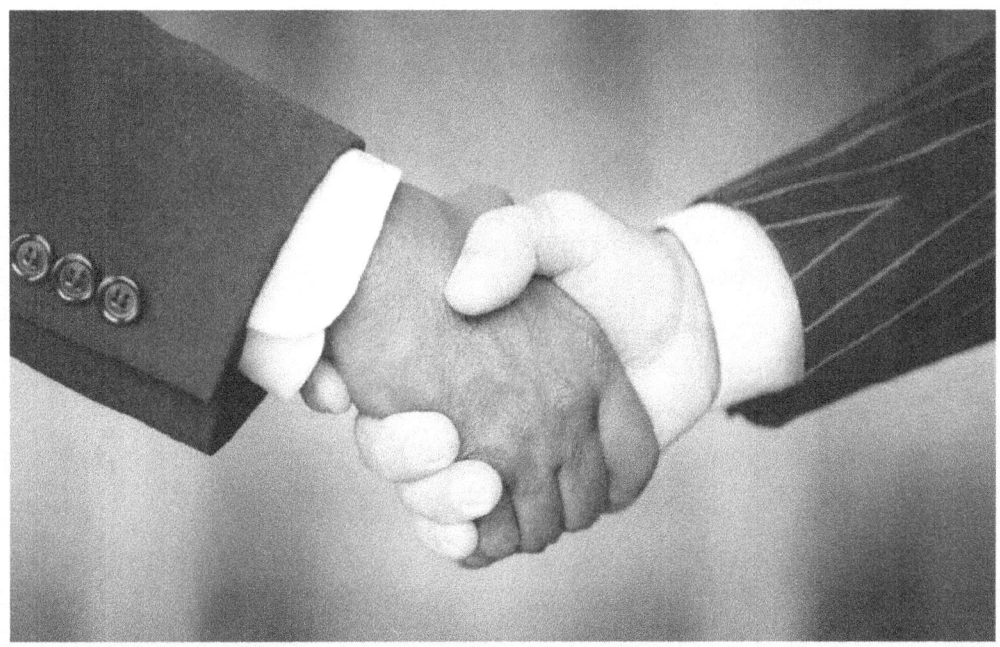

- Coalition and program promotion.
- Informing legislators and other stakeholders to gain support.
- Survivor and oncology events.
- Web site.
- Weekly governor's report.
- Press releases.

Success stories can be useful for marketing your program and gaining support for your efforts. They explain the important work being done in comprehensive cancer control and recognize the accomplishments of those working to improve cancer outcomes.

Stories should be interesting, easy to read, and relevant to the intended audience. To learn how to develop a compelling success story, see page 46 for helpful resources.

TABLE OF CONTENTS

EMPHASIZE PRIMARY PREVENTION OF CANCER

A person's cancer risk can be reduced by receiving regular medical care, avoiding tobacco, limiting alcohol use, avoiding excessive exposure to ultraviolet rays from the sun and tanning beds, eating a diet rich in fruits and vegetables, maintaining a healthy weight, and being physically active. Find out more at http://www.cdc.gov/cancer/dcpc/prevention.

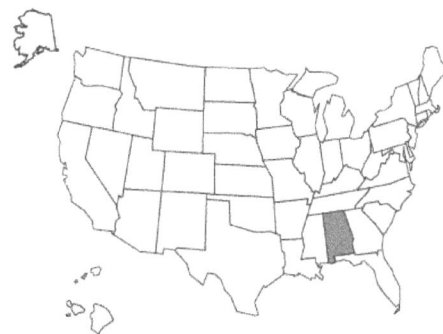

ALABAMA

"Third Time's the Charm" Campaign for HPV Vaccination

Human papillomavirus (HPV) is known to cause several types of cancer in both men and women. The virus, which is spread through sexual contact, is the leading cause of cervical cancer in women, with roughly 11,000 new cases and 4,000 deaths among U.S. women each year.*

The HPV vaccine is readily available and is a relatively easy way to prevent cervical cancer, yet only about half of teenage girls in the United States have taken the vaccine. One of the main reasons for skipping vaccination comes down to the sexual connotation attached to the virus—a barrier which has proven difficult to overcome.

In 2011, the Alabama Department of Public Health's (ADPH) Comprehensive Cancer Control Program joined with the ADPH Breast and Cervical Cancer Early Detection Program to create and carry out a campaign to promote HPV vaccination. The "Third Time's the Charm" campaign targets Alabama parents, physicians, and college students with a message that emphasizes the importance of getting all three doses of the HPV vaccine.

Parents and physicians are urged to begin the vaccinations at age 11, when it can be paired with the tetanus–diphtheria–pertussis vaccination, which is for Alabama's rising 6th-grade children. These vaccines are covered by most insurance plans and by the Vaccines for Children Program, managed by the Centers for Disease Control and Prevention. College students are reminded that under health care reform, the vaccines may be covered by their parents' insurance.

Campaign materials, including postcards, posters, and a 30-second commercial that ran in Alabama movie theaters throughout the

CONTACT

Alabama Comprehensive Cancer Control Program

■ 201 Monroe Street, Suite 1400-G
  Montgomery, AL 36130–3017

■ 800-252-1818

■ http://www.adph.org/cancercontrol

---

*U.S. Cancer Statistics Working Group. *United States Cancer Statistics: 1999–2008 Incidence and Mortality Web-based Report*. Atlanta: U.S. Department of Health and Human Services, Centers for Disease Control and Prevention and National Cancer Institute; 2012. Available at http://www.cdc.gov/uscs.

summer, were part of the campaign. These materials were adapted for a series of print ads running in parenting magazines and a journal for physicians.

After this initial push, the campaign has been working with the ADPH Immunization Division to send birthday cards with reminders about getting vaccines, including the HPV vaccine, to parents of Alabama girls on their 11th and 12th birthdays. "Third Time's the Charm" campaign materials have been expanded to include signs placed on gas pumps throughout Alabama and a small bracelet charm packaged with HPV educational material for college students.

REACH, a program created by CDC to eliminate racial and ethnic disparities in health care, contacted the Alabama Comprehensive Cancer Control Program about the possibility of using teen educators to speak to peers about the HPV virus and vaccine. They recognized the campaign as being particularly effective because it de-emphasizes the sexually transmitted disease portion of the message and concentrates instead on the virus's link to cervical cancer.

The "Third Time's the Charm" campaign addresses several barriers, particularly in educating residents and providers about the importance of getting all three doses of the vaccine. By emphasizing the virus's connection to cervical cancer, the campaign seeks to overcome the stigma associated with HPV vaccination in the minds of parents of young girls. The campaign has mailed more than 3,600 birthday cards each month to parents of 11-year-old girls and distributed close to 2,500 HPV information cards with an attached charm to college students. REACH has distributed 500 informational pamphlets and 1,000 "Third Time's the Charm" bookmarks to teen educators and community partners in the Birmingham area. Future plans include examining HPV immunization rates across the state to determine the effect of the campaign.

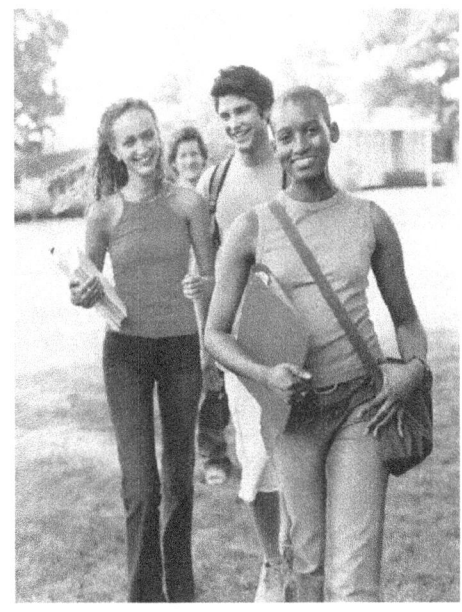

**Adding It Up:
Third Time's a Charm
Materials in the Community**

- *3,600 birthday cards*

- *2,500 HPV information cards*

- *1,000 bookmarks*

- *500 informational pamphlets*

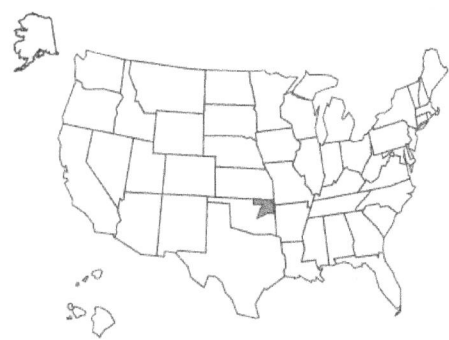

CHEROKEE NATION
Tobacco Tour Soon to Reach 5,000 School Kids

Although tobacco use among Cherokee Nation high school students seems to be dropping, many young people still take that first puff or dip and become habitual users. Studies show that nearly 90% of smokers begin before the age of 18, and 99% by the age of 26.*

In November 2008, the Cherokee Nation Comprehensive Cancer Control Program started the *Tobacco Tour*, which tells young people about the dangers of tobacco use. At first, it was aimed at fifth- to eighth-grade students, but has grown to include high school students.

The program presentation teaches students how nonceremonial tobacco use can lead to cancer and other health problems, but does not condemn the traditional use of tobacco for sacred American Indian ceremonies. The underlying theme of the program is that the choices students make now can affect their lives in the future. If they choose to use commercial tobacco, drugs, or alcohol, they may not be able to reach their life goals.

Next, eight-time Guinness World Record holder Brian Jackson tells about his life and the bad choices he made as a teen. He illustrates his story by making balloon animals and, at the end of his presentation, demonstrates one of his world records by making a hot water bottle burst using only his lungs.

The last presenter is Ronnie Trentham, a six-time cancer survivor, former smokeless tobacco user, and mayor of Stilwell, Oklahoma. He tells the kids he started chewing tobacco as a teen because all his

CONTACT

Cherokee Nation Comprehensive Cancer Control

■ PO Box 948
   Tahlequah, OK 74465
■ 800-256-0671
■ http://cancer.cherokee.org

*U.S. Department of Health and Human Services. Preventing Tobacco Use Among Youth and Young Adults [Fact Sheet]. Available at http://www.surgeongeneral.gov/library/reports/preventing-youth-tobacco-use/factsheet.html.

friends did it. He chewed tobacco for only 6 years, but believes it caused cancer in his jaw. He drives the point home with pictures of the surgery to remove his jawbone and the radiation treatments that followed. The pictures grab the kids' attention, but one draws an even bigger reaction. It is called "the Hairy Tongue" and has taste buds that have become precancerous cells, resembling a patch of dead grass.

At the end of the presentation, kids are told to look at their sphere of influence. These three talented and positive men show what people can achieve by making the right personal choices.

The *Tobacco Tour* message has been delivered to more than 4,400 students in 28 elementary schools in the Cherokee Nation's 14-county Tribal Jurisdictional Service Area in northeastern Oklahoma.

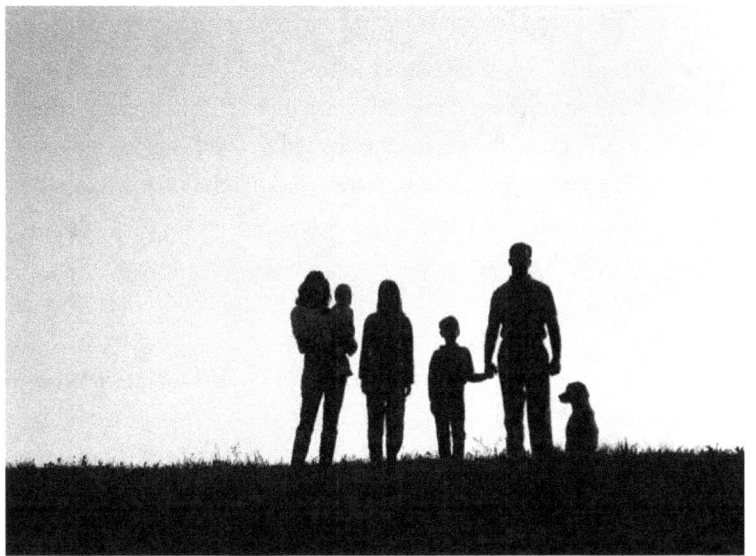

The 1½-hour presentation starts with Robert Lewis telling traditional Cherokee stories taught to him by tribal elders. With audience participation, he demonstrates the story he is telling. Each story is significant to Cherokee culture and easily ties into the antitobacco message.

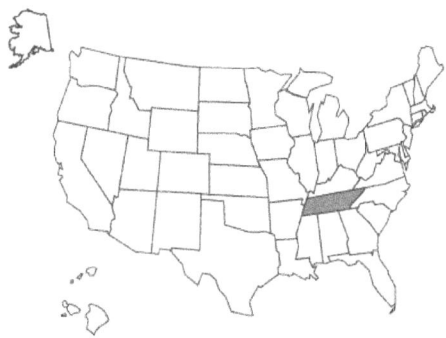

TENNESSEE

Tennessee Success Story

Obesity is a growing problem among children throughout the United States. In Tennessee, more than one-third of children aged 10–17 years are overweight or obese—the fourth highest rate in the nation. In addition, 23% of all deaths in Tennessee in 2005 were caused by cancer.*

In response, the Tennessee Comprehensive Cancer Control Program collaborated with Middle Tennessee State University to develop the A-B-C-1-2-3 Healthy Kids in Tennessee: Let's Eat Well, Play, and Be Aware Every Day program. Designed for child care providers, parents, and children aged 3–5 years, the program helps both children and adults understand the connection between lifestyle choices and chronic disease.

To participate in the A-B-C-1-2-3 program, child care facilities must offer educational opportunities for parents, children, and other family members for each area in the curriculum over the course of 12 weeks. These may include newsletters and handouts, workshops or presentations, and interactive classroom activities for the children. Facilities also receive information about selected topics, suggested activities, incentive gifts to share with parents and children, and volunteer presentations. Each class should do at least 30 minutes of active play or fitness at least three times per week and a nutrition activity for 10–15 minutes twice per week.

To help evaluate the program, child care providers fill out short surveys to assess their knowledge of physical activity, nutrition, and tobacco exposures; children wear pedometers to measure physical activity; parents answer questionnaires about their child's diet; and children's height and weight are measured before and after the program.

CONTACT

Tennessee Comprehensive Cancer Control Coalition

■ Cordell Hull Building, 6th Floor
425 Fifth Avenue North
Nashville, TN 37243

■ 615-741-1638

■ http://health.state.tn.us/CCCP

*Centers for Disease Control and Prevention. Tennessee: Burden of Chronic Diseases. Available at: http://www.cdc.gov/chronicdisease/states/pdf/tennessee.pdf.

The A-B-C-1-2-3 program is widening its reach through collaboration with the Tennessee Department of Health's Gold Sneakers initiative, which works to enhance policies related to physical activity, nutrition, and tobacco avoidance in licensed child care facilities. Together, they provide guidance for child care facilities to implement policy change and resources to facilitate healthy activities.

Through a partnership with the Tennessee Department of Human Services (DHS) and the Tennessee Child Care Resource and Referral Network, the voluntary Star-Quality program recognizes child care facilities that meet certain criteria with as many as three stars. Facilities that earn all three stars receive additional funding from the DHS.

Child care facilities may earn stars through the A-B-C-1-2-3 program. The director and staff members of participating child care centers can receive initial and ongoing training. A new Web site for the A-B-C-1-2-3 program will offer DHS-approved training credits to staff members at more than 700 child care facilities in the state.

It's never too early to start teaching children about healthy lifestyles. These efforts reach Tennessee's youngest residents and their caregivers to promote healthy living for the rest of their lives.

Research has shown that being overweight or obese raises a person's risk of getting endometrial (uterine), breast, and colorectal cancers.

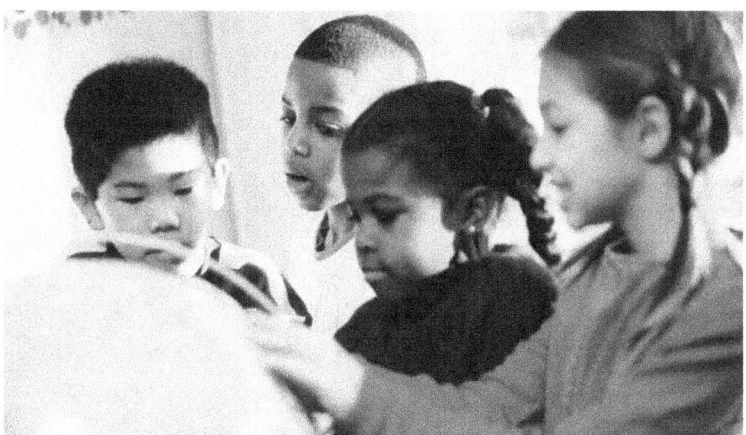

SUPPORT EARLY DETECTION AND TREATMENT ACTIVITIES

Screening means checking your body for cancer before you have symptoms. Getting screening tests regularly may find breast, cervical, and colorectal (colon) cancers early, when treatment is likely to work best. CDC supports screening for breast, cervical, and colorectal (colon) cancers as recommended by the U.S. Preventive Services Task Force. Find out more at http://www.ahrq.gov/clinic/uspstfix.htm.

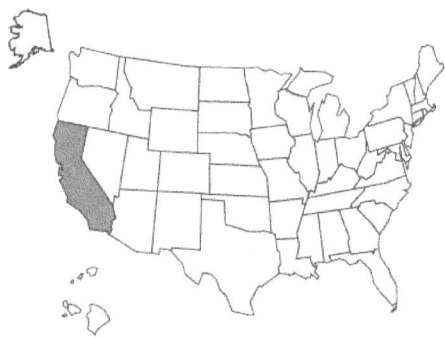

CALIFORNIA

Increasing Ovarian Cancer Awareness in California

Ovarian cancer is the fifth leading cause of cancer death among American women.* Each year, about 22,000 women in the United States are diagnosed with ovarian cancer, and about 15,000 women die from it.* Since there is no screening test for ovarian cancer (the Pap test checks for cervical cancer only), recognizing symptoms is crucial to diagnosing ovarian cancer early.

Until recently, ovarian cancer awareness advocates in California worked in local communities and had little communication with other groups. On June 26, 2009, 20 ovarian cancer survivors and founders of 16 local groups met to share ideas. This group became the California Ovarian Cancer Network.

A few months later, the network's Web site was launched to share information about local ovarian cancer resources and to draw attention to ovarian cancer efforts statewide. On August 15, 2010, California's first conference for ovarian cancer advocates, survivors, and medical professionals took place in Sacramento. The conference, Teal Impact: New Hopes and Future Directions, was named for the ovarian cancer awareness color, teal. Information was presented on the latest research and clinical trials, and attendees shared experiences. More than 80 people, including 38 ovarian cancer survivors, came to the conference.

A year after the Web site launched, a survey revealed a gap in member interaction. "The Web site is a good information-sharing tool for the public," members said, "but we also want to stay in touch with each other more regularly." As a result, a social networking site was built in May 2011. Through this social network, members can talk

CONTACT

California Comprehensive Cancer Control Program

■ 1825 Bell Street, Suite 102
Sacramento, CA 95825

■ 916-779-2611

■ http://www.cdph.ca.gov/programs/csrb/
Pages/default.aspx

*U.S. Cancer Statistics Working Group. *United States Cancer Statistics: 1999–2008 Incidence and Mortality Web-based Report.* Atlanta: U.S. Department of Health and Human Services, Centers for Disease Control and Prevention and National Cancer Institute; 2012. Available at http://www.cdc.gov/uscs.

to each other, post information about resources and upcoming events, upload photos, and customize a Web page for a local group.

New content attracts people to social media, so the network started an Ambassadorial Scholarship Program to enlist three members to take the lead in posting new content and inviting others to visit the site. The scholarship program also allowed the three ambassadors to travel to the Ovarian Cancer National Alliance Annual Conference in Washington, D.C., where they officially represented the network, found ways to work with other groups, and learned about the latest developments in ovarian cancer research and advocacy. When they returned to California, each ambassador posted conference reports and photos on the Web site.

The California Ovarian Cancer Network has grown from a small group to a network that connects advocates all over the state in just a few years. Member collaboration will be vital to increase early detection and treatment of ovarian cancer.

Ovarian cancer causes more deaths than any other cancer of the female reproductive system. But when ovarian cancer is found in its early stages, treatment is most effective.

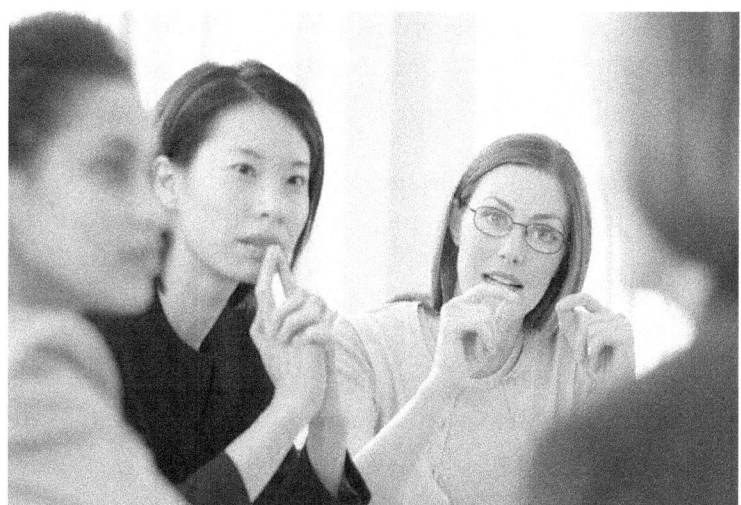

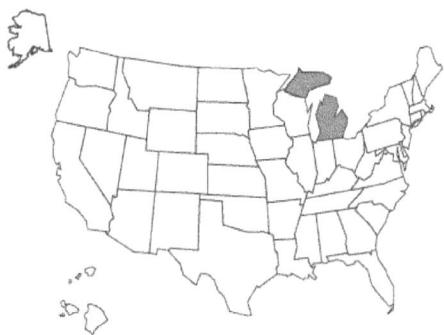

MICHIGAN

Cancer Screening of Underserved Women in Southeast Michigan

While rates of cervical cancer in the United States and Michigan have fallen significantly since the introduction of the Pap test, as many as 70% of women who die from cervical cancer either never had a Pap test or did not have one in the 5 years before getting cancer. Many women who get cervical cancer are older, are members of minority groups, and are unlikely to have regular health care. Women who are less likely to have had a Pap test in the previous 3 years include women with low incomes and less than a high school education, or those aged 18–29 years or aged 72 or older.*

Pap tests are important because cervical cancer may not cause symptoms. Regular Pap tests with follow-up when needed can prevent most cervical cancers.

The University of Michigan Health System (UMHS), a member of the Michigan Cancer Consortium, started the Pap Test Screening 2011 program with many internal and external partners. On March 26, 2011, from 1:00–4:00 PM, 12 rooms at the UMHS clinic were used to perform a Pap test every 15 minutes. Twelve doctors volunteered to perform the tests and Cancer AnswerLine nurses booked the appointments. Women who were at least 21 years old, had not had a Pap test in the previous 2 years, and did not have medical coverage for a Pap test were eligible to participate.

The event cost only about $1,300, most of which was associated with printing flyers, producing mailings, and providing lunch for volunteers. Supplies, lab costs, doctor time, and pathology reports were donated.

That day, 103 women were screened. Most were aged 25–59 years, with a majority being in their 40s and 50s. About half of the women were members of racial or ethnic minorities, primarily

---

*Michigan Department of Community Health. (2011). Estimates for Risk Factors and Health Indicators State of Michigan: Selected Tables: Michigan Behavioral Risk Factor Survey 2010. Available at http://www.michigan.gov/documents/mdch/2010_MiBRFS_Standard_Tables_FINAL_350512_7.pdf.

CONTACT

Michigan Comprehensive Cancer Control Program

■ Capitol View Building
201 Townsend Street
Lansing, MI 48913

■ 517-373-3740

■ http://www.michigan.gov/mdch/0,1607,7-132-2940_2955_2975-13561--,00.html

African-American. UMHS Interpreter Services provided interpreters for two Spanish-speaking and two Chinese-speaking participants.

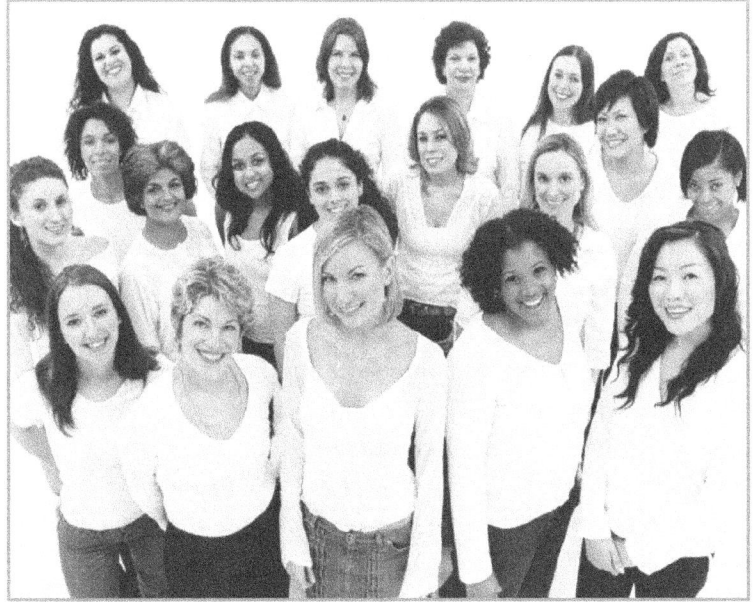

As many as 70% of women who die from cervical cancer either never had a Pap test or did not have one in the 5 years before getting cancer.

All women were given a list of local resources for free or low-cost health care, and health information including smoking cessation literature. Later, each woman received a letter with her test results. Seven women had abnormal results, and were contacted by a doctor or social worker for follow-up.

Sponsors learned several valuable lessons from the event. Scheduling the screening in a warmer month drew more registrants compared to the previous screening held in late January. Scheduling the event in the afternoon worked well, and efficiency was improved by having more clinic rooms available. However, a larger, earlier media push would have increased awareness and filled available appointments, and more Spanish-language health education materials were needed.

This successful model was repeated, thanks to funds from Verizon to carry out five Pap test screening days from the fall of 2011 to the fall of 2012.

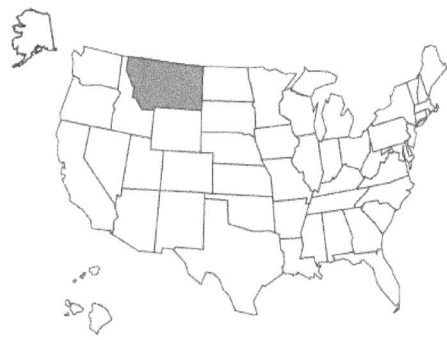

MONTANA

Colorectal Cancer Screening Among Insured Montanans

Though 82% of Montanans have health insurance that pays for colorectal cancer (CRC) screening, screening rates in Montana remain lower than the national average of 65%.* The Montana Cancer Control Program (MCCP) began educating insured adults aged ≥50 years about the importance of CRC screening, and letting them know that their health insurance plans cover the tests. The MCCP and the Montana Comprehensive Cancer Control Coalition set a priority to increase CRC screening rates across the state.

The MCCP began communicating with small employer association plans, groups that have private benefit packages for their members through the state's largest insurers. These plans were receptive to educating their members about the screening tests covered under their benefits packages and, also, about other covered preventive health services, including breast and cervical cancer screening.

MCCP's first partner organization was Insure Montana, a small employer purchasing pool that covers about 5,000 people, including 1,900 who are aged ≥50 years. Insure Montana provided baseline CRC screening rates for these members, and will provide these data for 3 years for evaluation purposes.

Over the course of about 6 months, MCCP

- Included a statement about CRC screening on each insured person's monthly assistance check.

- Included an article about colorectal cancer in the Insure Montana newsletter sent to everyone participating in the program.

- Targeted Insure Montana members aged ≥50 years who were not up-to-date on either a sigmoidoscopy or colonoscopy (about 1,200 members) and sent them a postcard about CRC screening and health insurance coverage for the test.

CONTACT

Montana Cancer Control Section

■ PO Box 202951
1400 Broadway, Room C317
Helena, MT 59620-2951

■ 406-444-6089

■ http://www.dphhs.mt.gov/publichealth/
cancer/comprehensivecancercontrolplan.
shtml

---

*Montana Census and Economic Information Center. Montana Behavioral Risk Factor Surveillance Survey 2010. Available at http://ceic.mt.gov/MtByNumb.asp.

As MCCP developed its partnership with Insure Montana, they approached several other organizations. All of these organizations shared their members' CRC screening rates as part of the evaluation plan. Outreach activities included efforts such as postcard reminders with each organization's information on insurance coverage available for these services. This was also a great opportunity to educate members about changes to insurance coverage for preventive services that the Affordable Care Act[†] will bring. Through these campaigns, MCCP reached about 92,000 Montanans—almost 10% of the state's population.

In addition to working directly with insuring organizations and employers, MCCP has worked with It Starts With Me (ISWM) (http://www.itstartswithme.com), a company that provides wellness screening for many partners. MCCP and ISWM have developed a personalized message for participants aged ≥50 years who receive wellness screenings through their employers. The message is included in the screening results provided to participants and explains the importance of age-appropriate cancer screening and what insurance coverage is available.

This project has helped MCCP to build relationships with insurers and employers. They also are working with their partners on breast and cervical cancer screening messages, as well as integrated chronic disease prevention programs.

The U.S. Preventive Services Task Force recommends colorectal cancer screening for men and women aged 50–75 using high-sensitivity fecal occult blood testing, sigmoidoscopy, or colonoscopy.

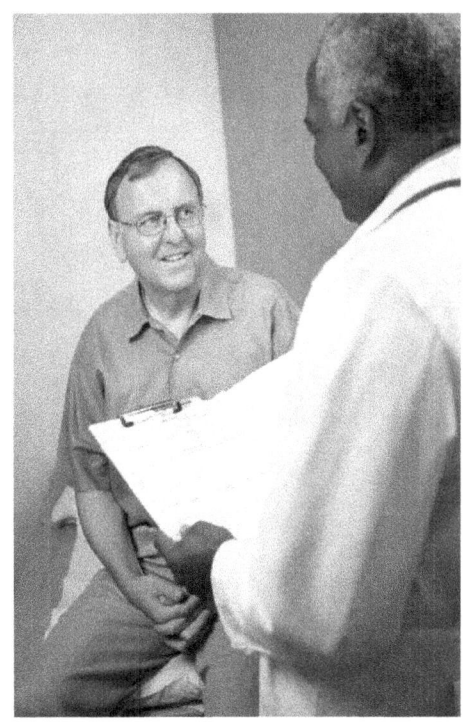

[†]Koh HK, Sebelius KG. Promoting Prevention through the Affordable Care Act. *New England Journal of Medicine* 2010;363:1293–1299. Available at http://www.nejm.org/doi/full/10.1056/NEJMp1008560.

ADDRESS PUBLIC HEALTH NEEDS OF CANCER SURVIVORS

A *cancer survivor* is a person who has been diagnosed with cancer, from the time of diagnosis throughout his or her life. To reduce the impact of this increasing burden of cancer, medical and public health professionals need to address possible long-term and late effects of cancer and its treatment on survivors' physical and psychosocial well-being, provide them with coordinated care, and promote healthy behaviors. Find out more at http://www.cdc.gov/cancer/survivorship/what_cdc_is_doing/research/survivors_article.htm.

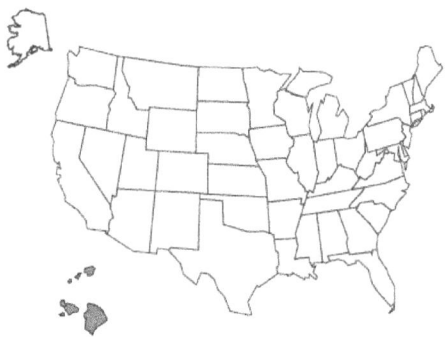

HAWAII

Journey Together: The Quality of Life Cancer Survivorship Conference

One hundred years ago, people with cancer had little hope of long-term survival. Today, when normal life expectancy is taken into consideration, about two of every three cancer patients are alive 5 years after diagnosis.

In Hawaii, the number of people who were diagnosed with cancer increased from 1975 to 2005, though incidence remained fairly stable and death rates dropped. This means more people are living longer after a cancer diagnosis. As a result, survivorship and quality of life issues have become more important.

One of the goals of the Hawaii State Cancer Plan is to improve the quality of life of cancer survivors. The Hawaii Comprehensive Cancer Control Coalition's (HCCCC) Quality of Life Action Team worked with many partners statewide to address this goal. The team included cancer survivors, patient navigators, national partners, hospitals, and community organizations. Monthly meetings were held to learn what survivors need.

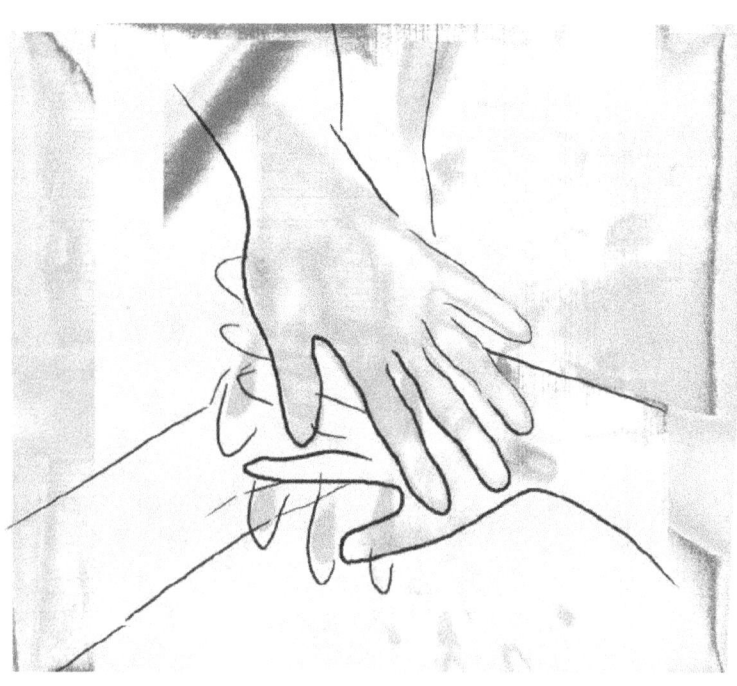

CONTACT

Hawai'i Comprehensive Cancer Control Program

■ 601 Kamokila Blvd., Room 344
Kapolei, HI 96707

■ 808-692-7480

■ http://hawaii.gov/health/family-child-health/
chronic-disease/cccp/index.html

The team hosted the Journey Together: The Quality of Life Cancer Survivorship Conference on the island of Oahu to bring cancer survivors and caregivers together to discuss life after cancer treatment. Combining funds with partner organizations, the team offered scholarships for participants from neighboring islands to come to the conference.

In all, 206 survivors, caregivers, nurses, cancer support group members, patient navigators, community cancer partners, and family members attended the conference. In addition to the conference, 125 conference attendees participated in a pre-symposium featuring leading experts speaking on promising cancer research, new cancer therapies, and how science has improved survival.

Feedback from conference attendees was extremely positive. Based on evaluation forms (60% return rate), attendees had high ratings for all eight panel sessions, including aspects of the conference such as how knowledgeable the presenters were and overall quality of presentations.

The HCCCC Quality of Life Action Team gave the evaluations to the planning committee and key partners, who will use the information to create topics for the next annual cancer survivorship conference. Respondents indicated other areas of interest for future conferences, including

- "Need presentations focusing on younger cancer survivors and the mental and physical effects of diagnosis, chemotherapy, and sexuality."

- "More information on clinical trials. Individuals either don't know about it or don't understand the process."

- "There is much more that must be done to increase survivorship and address the psychosocial needs of cancer patients and their families."

Attendees voiced a definite need for annual events such as the conference to provide cancer survivorship resources, hope, and inspiration for the people and families in Hawaii affected by cancer. The HCCCC Quality of Life Action Team has already started planning for next year's annual survivorship conference.

"Presenters were fabulous!"

"Was a very eye-opening, educational experience for me. The presenters were extremely knowledgeable and well spoken."

"Very well done by a nurse who knows what she is talking about!"

"Just a lot of helpful, useful information that applies directly to my situation."

"Learned from each presentation. Met many survivors of 10 years. Gives one much hope."

—Feedback from Quality of Life Cancer Survivorship Conference Attendees

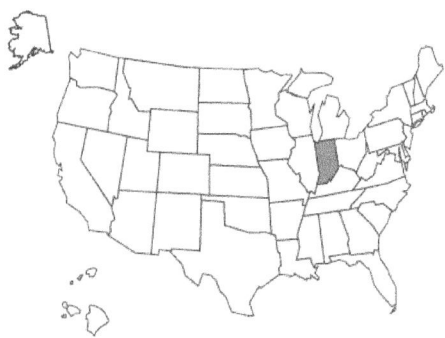

INDIANA

The Hoosier Cancer Story: Using Media to Promote, Educate, and Inspire

Across Indiana, cancer stories are common. The unfortunate truth is that any Hoosier seeking a cancer story could simply call a family member or neighbor.

Cancer is the second leading cause of death in Indiana. The four most frequently diagnosed cancers in Indiana from 2003–2007 were lung, colorectal, breast, and prostate. During 2003–2007, Indiana had among the highest rates of lung, female breast, and colorectal cancer deaths in the United States.*

As health professionals, it is our responsibility to lead the fight against cancer with solid research, proven policy, and effective interventions; in Indiana, we want to go a step further. In 2010, the Indiana Cancer Consortium (ICC) began sharing cancer stories with the release of the Indiana Cancer Control Plan (ICCP) 2010–2014 (http://indianacancer.org/indiana-cancer-control-plan/). The ICC is a network of public and private partnerships whose mission is to reduce the burden of cancer in Indiana across the continuum from prevention through pain management.

The ICCP consists of six focus areas, with one goal per focus area: primary prevention, early detection, treatment, quality of life, data, and advocacy. Results of a survey to identify gaps in plan implementation showed that member organizations were implementing all of the 250+ evidence-based strategies outlined in the ICCP.

CONTACT

Indiana Comprehensive Cancer Control Program

■ 2 North Meridian Street, 6B
   Indianapolis, IN 46204

■ 410-767-0750

■ http://www.in.gov/isdh/24969.htm

*U.S. Cancer Statistics Working Group. *United States Cancer Statistics: 1999–2008 Incidence and Mortality Web-based Report*. Atlanta: U.S. Department of Health and Human Services, Centers for Disease Control and Prevention and National Cancer Institute; 2012. Available at http://www.cdc.gov/uscs.

Ongoing evaluations indicate not only improved communication with partners, but also greater interest in ICC membership, programming, and policies. The Web site has seen a constant increase in visitors; information about ICC and full stories of 16 cancer survivors can be found at http://www.indianacancer.org. ICC membership has grown, and a weekly e-mail newsletter, an ICC Twitter account, and the ICC Facebook page share stories with ICC members and partners from health and media organizations, cancer survivors, health professionals, and residents in Indiana and nationwide.

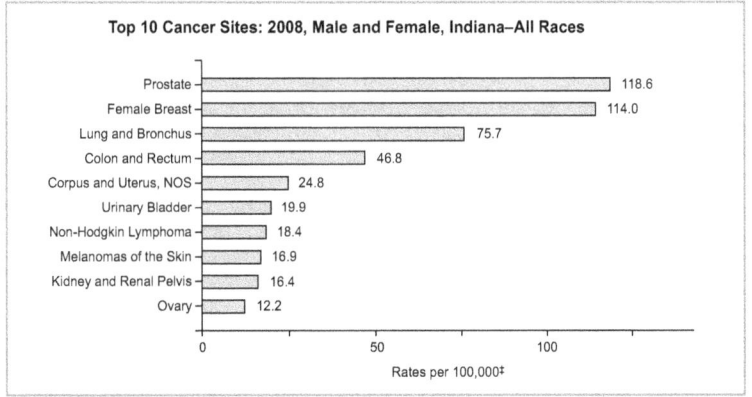

The path to success in Indiana has never been clearer: reduce the cancer burden by making it much harder to find tragic cancer stories. The task is no small feat but, as lung cancer survivor Molly Wooldridge so eloquently states, "No one should ever go from this world without a fight, even though it may be one of the hardest battles you've ever fought." Well, Hoosiers are fighting, and the ICC vows to continue sharing their stories.

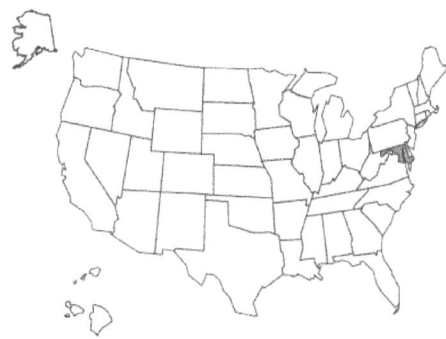

MARYLAND

Maryland Forum Honors and Educates Cancer Survivors

Each year, more than 24,000 Marylanders are diagnosed with invasive cancer. About 7% of adults in Maryland were cancer survivors in 2009 and, as death rates decrease, the number of cancer survivors increases.*

Cancer survivors deal with many difficult issues, including getting lifesaving and evidence-based cancer care, as well as care for treatment-related side effects and mental health problems. Many of the stresses cancer survivors face can be reduced or eliminated with the help of mental health, legal, and financial services; peer support networks; and patient education conferences.

As better treatment slows the progress of cancer, more people are living longer as survivors. However, resources and support are needed to help them maintain their quality of life after cancer. In addition to the direct cost of medical care and wages lost due to illness, cancer patients must pay for related expenses such as high insurance deductibles, transportation to treatment, and mental health services.

The Maryland Comprehensive Cancer Control Plan (MCCCP) has a goal of enhancing cancer survivors' quality of life through information and supportive services. Many strategies address this goal, including the organization of a statewide event to celebrate National Cancer Survivors Day and raise awareness about survivors' needs.

CONTACT

Maryland Comprehensive Cancer Control Program

■ 201 West Preston Street, 4th Floor, Suite 400
Baltimore, MD 21201-2399

■ 410-767-0750

■ http://fha.dhmh.maryland.gov/cancer/cancerplan/SitePages/Home.aspx

*Maryland Department of Health and Mental Hygiene. Center for Cancer Surveillance and Control. Available at http://fha.dhmh.maryland.gov/cancer/SitePages/Home.aspx.

On June 4, 2011, more than 300 people—including more than 200 cancer survivors—gathered in Baltimore, Maryland for Beyond Cancer: A Cancer Survivorship Forum. The forum was the result of a partnership between the MCCCP and the Prevention and Research Center at Mercy Medical Center, organized to honor National Cancer Survivors Day and provide education about survivorship issues.

The forum featured presentations about survivorship trends and research, offered practical take-home information, and gave survivors an opportunity to connect with one another. One keynote speaker focused on survivorship care and research; the other focused on the cancer experience from a patient's perspective. Activities to help with emotional well-being included a demonstration by a representative from a Buddhist center in Baltimore on the benefits of mindful meditation and a workshop on stress reduction and music therapy.

Other workshop topics included managing treatment side effects, complementary medicine, legal and insurance issues, balancing work and life after treatment, exercise and nutrition, and genetic testing. The forum ended with a cancer survivor reception.

The forum educated participants about cancer survivors' needs. According to participant evaluation forms, participants' knowledge increased by 26%, the overall forum was rated 4.7 out of 5, and all presenters received effectiveness scores of very good or higher. The positive feedback shows that large educational survivorship programs are both necessary and effective. The MCCCP hopes to repeat the forum annually as part of a larger awareness campaign around National Cancer Survivors Day.

As death rates decrease, the number of cancer survivors increases. In 2009, about 7% of Maryland adults were cancer survivors.

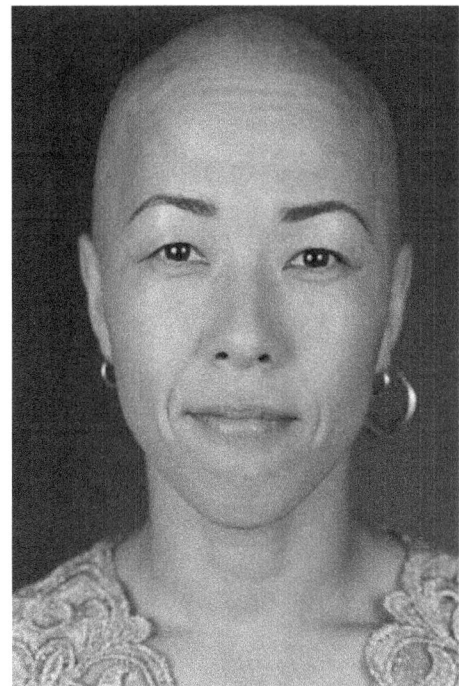

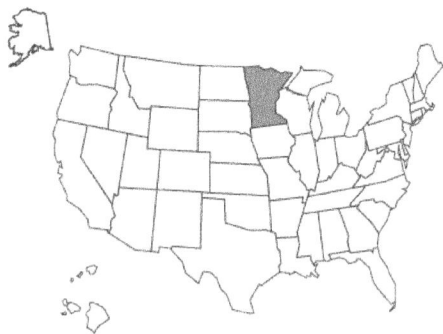

MINNESOTA

Promoting Continuity of Care for Cancer Survivors in Minnesota

The transition from active cancer treatment to survivorship is difficult. Many health care providers are not aware of the challenges facing survivors as they complete their treatment. At a time when survivors are expected to feel successful and healthy, many face physical and emotional reminders of their treatment.

In 2008, a group of Minnesota Cancer Alliance (MCA) members gathered to start a project to address the needs of cancer survivors. They wanted to improve continuity of care for cancer patients—to help bridge the transition from active patient care to life beyond cancer treatment. One of the key recommendations in the Institute of Medicine's report, *From Cancer Patient to Cancer Survivor: Lost in Transition** was that "the National Cancer Institute, professional associations, and voluntary organizations should expand and coordinate their efforts to provide educational opportunities to health care providers to equip them to address the health care and quality of life issues facing cancer survivors." [page 354]

Inspired by this recommendation, the MCA group envisioned an interdisciplinary conference to educate health care providers about the special needs of cancer survivors. MCA member organizations and the National Cancer Institute sponsored the meeting. Other member organizations made donations totaling more than $23,000. Several national comprehensive cancer control partners were involved in the development and success of the conference, including LIVE**STRONG**, the National Coalition for Cancer Survivors, the American Cancer Society, and the Patient Advocate Foundation.

CONTACT

Minnesota Comprehensive Cancer Control Program

■ 717 Delaware Street SE
Minneapolis, MN 55414

■ 651-201-3605

■ http://www.health.state.mn.us/divs/hpcd/compcancer/index.html

*Institute of Medicine. *From Cancer Patient to Cancer Survivor: Lost in Transition.* Washington: National Academy of Sciences; 2005. Available at http://iom.edu/Reports/2005/From-Cancer-Patient-to-Cancer-Survivor-Lost-in-Transition.aspx.

The conference, Bridging the Transition to Life after Cancer Treatment, was held April 29–30, 2011 in Bloomington, Minnesota. More than 130 providers attended the conference, including 20 physicians, 28 nurses, and 8 social workers. Most participants came from Minnesota, but the audience included residents of eight other states, from as far away as Alaska.

Featured speakers included Dr. Patricia Ganz, a nationally recognized physician and cancer survivorship researcher from the University of California, Los Angeles, who spoke about improving quality of care, and Dr. Jon Hallberg, a well-known Twin Cities-area family practice physician and media personality who used theater to explore the patient experience.

Conference breakout sessions were organized into three tracks: identifying, preventing, and managing comorbidities and treatment-related complications; lifestyle recommendations to prevent chronic disease among cancer survivors; and psychosocial, spiritual, and relationship issues after cancer treatment.

Many participants were inspired to use survivor care plans for their patients. They also wanted to implement, expand, or improve survivorship programs and services in their cancer centers and work with other health professionals to improve continuity of care.

The term "cancer survivor" refers to an individual who has been diagnosed with cancer, from the time of diagnosis throughout his or her life. The impact of cancer on family members, friends, and caregivers of survivors is also acknowledged as part of survivorship. Approximately 66% of people diagnosed with cancer are expected to live at least 5 years after diagnosis.

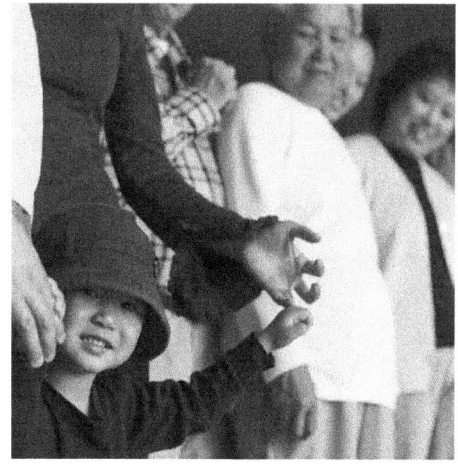

IMPLEMENT POLICY, SYSTEMS, AND ENVIRONMENTAL CHANGES TO GUIDE SUSTAINABLE CANCER CONTROL

Policy change is an increasingly effective way to control cancer. Public health is providing the evidence necessary to enhance the comprehensive cancer control agenda to implement effective policy, systems and environmental change strategies, and best practices at state and federal levels. Programs that have improved public health through policy change share their stories here.

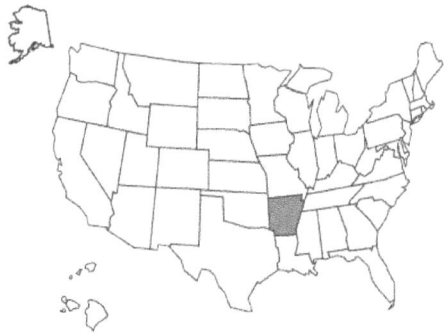

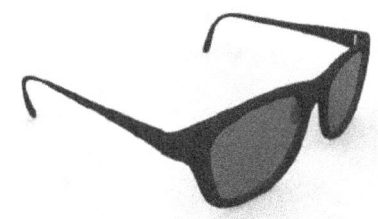

ARKANSAS
Inspiration and Collaboration Result in a Sun SMART Program

The Donald W. Reynolds Cancer Support House in Fort Smith, Arkansas, provides free nonmedical support programs and services to cancer patients and their families, and educational programs to the community. When staff members read the Arkansas Cancer Plan, they were alarmed to learn that new cases of melanoma, the deadliest kind of skin cancer, rose 53% between 1997 and 2007 in Arkansas. The Support House staff decided to help Arkansans protect themselves from skin cancer and created the Sun SMART program.

In a memorable way, the Sun SMART program helps people prevent skin cancer. SMART is an acronym for:

• **S**lip on a hat or T-shirt.

• **M**ove to the shade.

• **A**pply sunscreen with an SPF of at least 30.

• **R**eapply sunscreen every few hours.

• **T**ell your friends to be Sun SMART.

The Support House staff developed a campaign for the Sun SMART program, recruited partners to help get the message out, and found support including grants and sponsorships. This summer, the program will reach more than 5,000 kids with the Sun SMART message and provide lifeguard training, adult education, free skin cancer screenings, and gallons of sunscreen to swimmers at the city pool.

Fort Smith Parks Department
Support House is located across the street from the beautiful Creekmore Park so, from the beginning, staff knew it would be a perfect place to kick off the Sun SMART program. Kids were invited to the park where they watched Scudder the Amazing Frisbee Dog doing tricks and received gifts, frozen fruit treats, sunscreen samples,

CONTACT

Arkansas Comprehensive Cancer Control Program

■ 4815 West Markham Street
Little Rock, AR 72205

■ 800-462-0599

■ http://www.healthy.arkansas.gov/
programsServices/chronicDisease/
ComprehensiveCancerControl/Pages/
default.aspx

and Sun SMART education. They made crafts from UV beads that change color in the sun, and their fingernails were painted with UV polish. Now each summer, volunteers continue to get out the Sun SMART message at the park and the Sun SMART program keeps a sunscreen dispenser filled at the park's pool so swimmers will have access to sunscreen.

Fort Smith Public Library

At the Fort Smith Library, the 1,500 kids that participated in the summer reading program received a Sun SMART information card, sunscreen, and an invitation to join a Sun SMART story time. Each story time featured summer fun books, the Sun SMART message, a UV bead craft, and a snack.

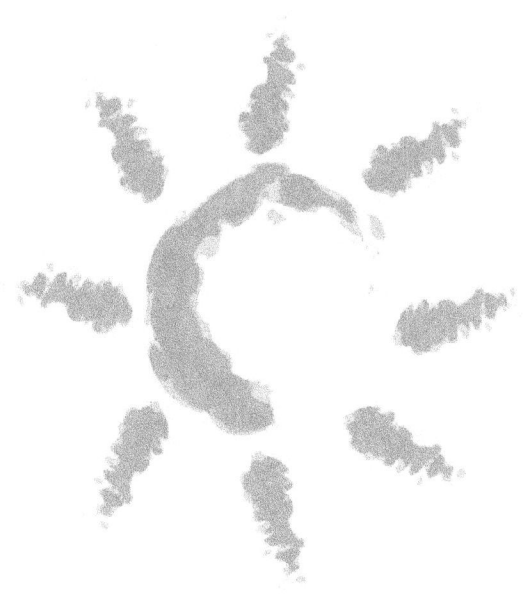

Protection from ultraviolet (UV) radiation is important all year round, not just during the summer or at the beach. UV rays from the sun can reach you on cloudy and hazy days, as well as bright and sunny days. UV rays also reflect off of surfaces like water, cement, sand, and snow.

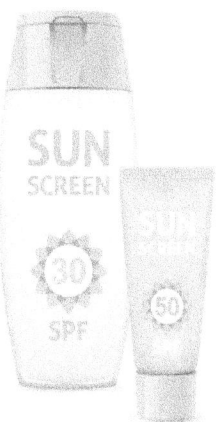

The Arkansas Cancer Plan at Work

Managed by the Arkansas Cancer Coalition, the Arkansas Cancer Plan shows what can be done for cancer prevention, detection, and care. The Sun SMART plan is a successful example of the Arkansas Cancer Plan at work. When they saw a need, Support House staff members found a creative way to deliver a cancer prevention message and also recruited partners to help deliver the message and fund the program.

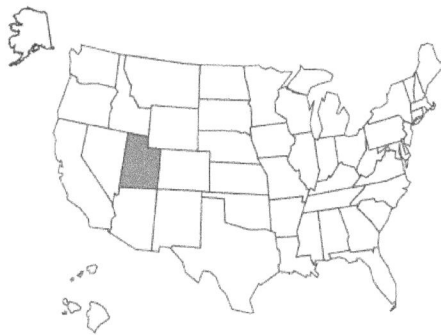

UTAH

Radon Education and Mitigation in Utah County

The United States Environmental Protection Agency (EPA) ranks radon among the top four environmental risks to Americans. Because there is no known safe level of exposure to radon, EPA recommends that those whose homes are in the highest radon potentials, Zone 1 and Zone 2, take steps to lessen radon levels.* The Utah Department of Environmental Quality (UDEQ) showed that 35% of the homes tested in Utah County were in Zone 1.

Builders in Utah are encouraged, though not required, to use radon-resistant construction in Zone 1 and Zone 2 areas, and there is a need for radon-resistant new construction techniques in Utah County. This is especially important considering the county's growth trends; about 1,200 new residential construction building permits were issued in 2009.

The Utah Department of Health's Comprehensive Cancer Control Program provides mini-grants to community organizations to support the Utah Comprehensive Cancer Prevention and Control Plan. Habitat for Humanity of Utah County (HHU) and the Utah County Health Department received a mini-grant to increase radon awareness among residents and show that radon reduction can be a part of all home building and renovating projects.

This project educated elementary-aged students, home builders, and inspectors on the dangers of radon; promoted radon testing; and worked with builders to apply radon-resistant techniques. They also contributed to building three new radon-resistant homes and decreasing radon in two renovation homes. The first radon-resistant

CONTACT

Utah Cancer Control Program

■ 288 North 1460 West
PO Box 142107
Salt Lake City, UT 84117-2107

■ 800-717-1811

■ http://www.cancerutah.org//About_UCCP/
Contact_Us.php

*United States Environmental Protection Agency. Radon. Available at http://www.epa.gov/radon.

home built was highlighted at a press conference on September 14, 2010 as part of the official kickoff for *Radon Tee: World Trek 2010*, a social media project sponsored by Cancer Survivors Against Radon (CanSAR) that used photos, videos, and personal stories to increase radon awareness, testing, and mitigation in communities around the world.

The project also

- Displayed information about radon testing and distributed about 100 radon test kits at the ReStore, HHU's resale outlets that sell reusable and surplus building materials to the public.

- Gave presentations at four elementary schools in Utah County to approximately 300 students and teachers about the link between indoor radon and lung cancer. Utah County students submitted about 60 posters to the National Radon Poster Contest.

- Provided a free continuing education course through UDEQ's Division of Radiation Control to 18 builders and inspectors who are members of the Utah Valley Home Builders Association.

These efforts have led to sustainable change in Utah County and throughout the state. UDEQ obtained funding from the EPA to have three HHU construction staff certified to install radon mitigation systems. HHU is committed to making all of their homes radon resistant because of the success of this project, and plans are underway to create a toolkit so that other builders can have similar results.

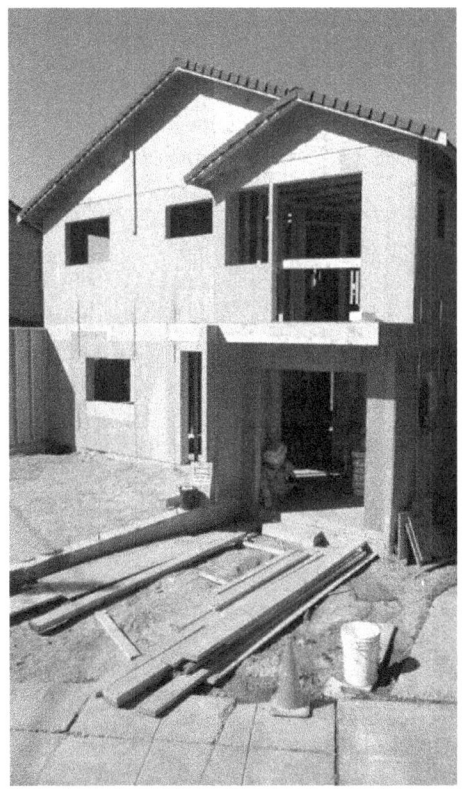

Radon is an odorless, colorless, radioactive gas. It is the second leading cause of lung cancer in the United States. Because radon comes from so many sources, people are easily exposed to it. Radon gas can seep through cracks in buildings and expose people to the radiation.

PROMOTE HEALTH EQUITY AS IT RELATES TO CANCER CONTROL

According to CDC's Office of Minority Health and Health Disparities, life expectancy and overall health have improved in recent years for most Americans. However, not all Americans are benefiting equally. CDC monitors trends and patterns in cancer incidence and mortality and identifies which populations are disproportionately affected by the disease. Find out more at http://www.cdc.gov/omhd.

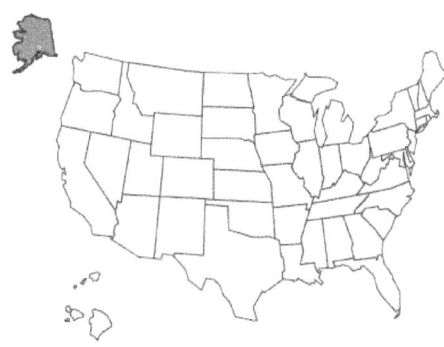

ALASKA NATIVE TRIBAL HEALTH CONSORTIUM

Alaska Native Men's Retreat for Prostate and Testicular Cancer Survivors

Prostate cancer is the most common kind of cancer in American men, with more than three out of four cases diagnosed in men over age 65.* The average age-adjusted incidence rates during 2004–2008 for prostate cancer in Alaska Native men was 66.4/100,000, compared to 153.0/100,000 in U.S. white men. Mortality rates for 1994–2008 also were lower for Alaska Native men than U.S. white men (19.0/100,000 vs. 27.0/100,000).[†]

Urinary, bowel, sexual, and hormonal problems are often side effects of prostate or testicular cancer treatment. These side effects can reduce survivors' physical, mental, and social well-being. Though cancer patient support groups reduce depression, men may choose not to join them because general support groups don't meet prostate and testicular cancer survivors' special needs.

In 2009, the Alaska Native Tribal Health Consortium (ANTHC) and the Alaska Comprehensive Cancer Control Program, in collaboration with the Alaska Prostate Cancer Collation and local clinics, started the annual Men's Retreat for Prostate and Testicular Cancer Survivors. Retreat activities included fishing, rafting, and hiking to attract men to the event, especially those who have never been part of a cancer support group.

Until 2011, the retreat was offered only in Cooper Landing, Alaska, near Anchorage. In 2011, with help from ANTHC and the Mayo Clinic, the South East Area Regional Health Consortium (SEARHC) held a men's retreat on Prince of Wales Island in Craig, Alaska.

> "A few men who attended actually called the SEARHC president and stopped by my office just to tell me how much they appreciated the opportunity to attend the retreat."

CONTACT

Alaska Native Tribal Health Consortium

■ 4000 Ambassador Drive
Anchorage, AK 99508

■ 907-729-1900

■ http://www.anthctoday.org

---

*U.S. Cancer Statistics Working Group. *United States Cancer Statistics: 1999–2008 Incidence and Mortality Web-based Report*. Atlanta: U.S. Department of Health and Human Services, Centers for Disease Control and Prevention; National Cancer Institute; 2012. Available at: http://www.cdc.gov/uscs.

†National Cancer Institute. Surveillance, Epidemiology and End Results (SEER) Program. Available at http://www.seer.cancer.gov.

This retreat was offered only to Alaska Native prostate cancer survivors living in southeast Alaska, which has few resources for survivors. The only other men's cancer support groups in Alaska, the Us Too prostate cancer support groups, are in south central Alaska at Anchorage and Soldotna.

In addition to providing sponsorship for the SEARHC's men's retreat, the Mayo Clinic sent a urologist and an internist to serve as expert advisors for the men throughout the weekend. ANTHC completed an evaluation of the retreat, which found that it was well received by the men and that they would recommend it to other survivors.

This joint effort between ANTHC and SEARHC demonstrated how an established program could be tailored to fit the needs of regional tribal health organizations and cancer survivors in rural areas.

Cooper Landing (South Central Alaska) All Races	
Year	Number of Participants
2009	16
2010	16
2011	17
Total	49

Prince of Wales Island (Southeast Alaska) Alaska Native Men Only	
Year	Number of Participants
2011	10
2012	10
Total	20

"One participant stopped by my office and handed me a handful of sponsor applications. He had actually gone around town and shared his men's retreat experience with the local tribes, corporations, and other businesses asking them for their support in future men's retreats. He then brought me the applications and told me he hopes to see this retreat continue."

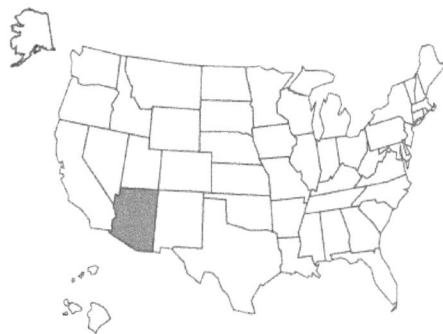

ARIZONA

In the Beginning

To enable local community cancer organizations and partners nationwide to increase services to cancer patients and their families, the Centers for Disease Control and Prevention funded the American Psychological Association's Socioeconomic Status Related Cancer Disparities (SESRCD) Program. One local organization, the Arizona Cancer Coalition, used the funding to award small grants to three programs to support activities emphasizing community partnerships.

The **Asian Pacific Community in Action (APCA)** received funding for a Native Hawaiian and other Pacific Islander Personal Digital Stories Project among residents in the Phoenix metropolitan area. Native Hawaiian women have the highest rate of uterine cancer in the nation, the second highest rate for all cancers combined, and the second highest rates for cancers of the lung, pancreas, and ovary. They also have the third highest breast cancer death rate.

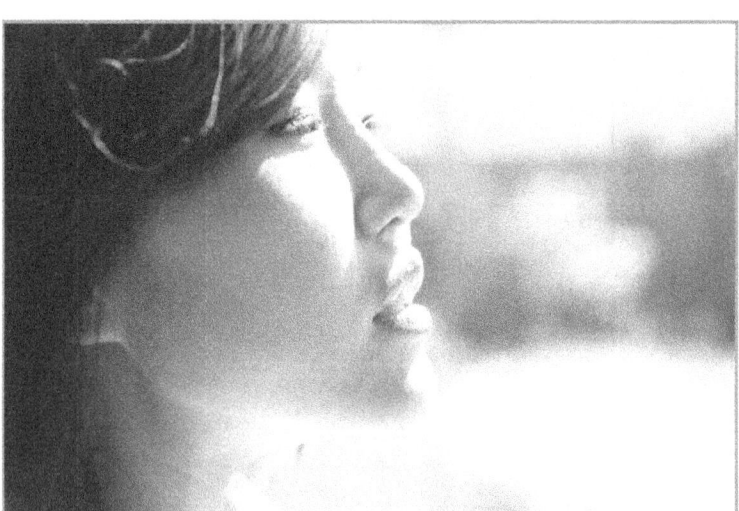

The APCA trained five cancer survivors from the local Chamorro community to write and share their personal digital stories. The stories focused on each survivor's cancer journey and the impact it had on them and their families. The stories were presented to the public and have been placed on the APCA Web site (http://www.apcaaz.org/women.htm).

CONTACT

Arizona Cancer Control Program

◼ 150 North 18th Avenue
  Suite 300
  Phoenix, AZ 85007

◼ 602-364-0824

◼ http://www.azdhs.gov/azcancercontrol

The **Arizona Myeloma Network** (AzMN) received funding for its third annual AzMN/Ft. Defiance Cancer Awareness and Advocacy Conference for the Navajo Nation. Cancer was the second leading cause of death among Navajos in 2004, and Navajo people have the lowest 5-year survival rate of any group in the country.* Translated in Navajo as the "sore that does not heal," cancer has been a taboo subject among Native people, who avoid speaking of the disease for fear of wishing it upon family and being rejected. The conference

- Increased cancer awareness, education, and advocacy.

- Provided resources to help patients and families make better treatment choices.

- Brought together new and existing services, including programs that help with earlier diagnosis, improve treatment, and provide better quality of life for cancer survivors and their families.

More than 330 cancer advocates attended the conference and learned much about local needs and solutions. Most attendees who were surveyed said the quality of the conference, speakers, and workshops was excellent or good, and they received information they could use and share with others.

The **Southwest Prostate Cancer Foundation (SWPCF)** received funding to broadcast a weekly radio show about cancer and other health issues, and to provide free prostate cancer screenings. Prostate cancer is the most common cancer in men and the second leading cause of death among men in Arizona.

The SWPCF created a network of speakers and developed the weekly radio show. It also worked with providers and health care organizations to provide free prostate cancer screenings.

In Navajo, "cancer" translates as "the sore that does not heal."

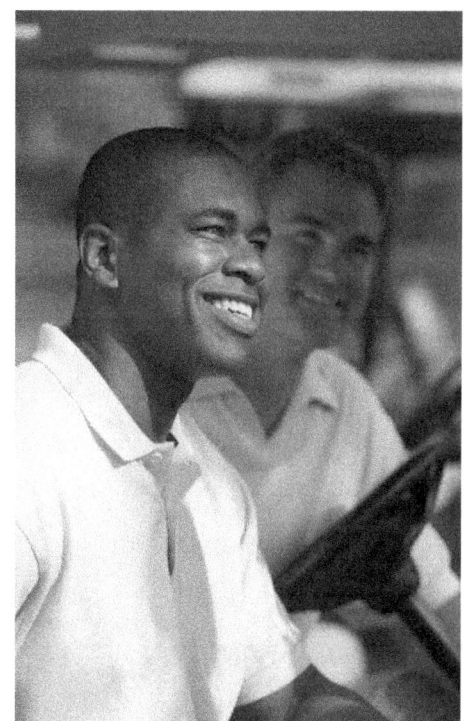

---

*Arizona Department of Health Services. Arizona Cancer Registry. Available at http://www.azdhs.gov/phs/phstats/acr/index.htm.

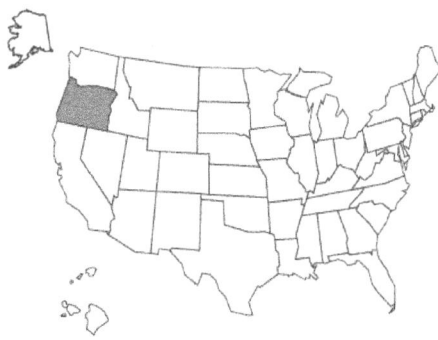

OREGON

Preventing Cancer Through Community Empowerment

Colorectal cancer (CRC) is the second most deadly cancer that affects both men and women, but it does not have to be. Screening can prevent CRC or catch it early when it is highly treatable. But too few men and women in Oregon have been screened.

The Oregon Partnership for Cancer Control (OPCC) started a new campaign to increase screening rates for CRC to 80% among people aged 50–75 years by 2014. In Oregon, CRC screening rates during 2006–2009 were 44.1%.

OPCC selected Clatsop County for a pilot study because the CRC death rate is significantly higher there than in the rest of the state (23/100,000 in Clatsop County versus 18/100,000 in Oregon overall). Six recognizable spokespeople from across Clatsop County who had been screened for CRC agreed to have their stories published in print, in campaign materials, on a Web site (http://www.TheCancerYouCanPrevent.org), and in radio ads. Their stories focused on the ease and importance of being screened and why people should get screened.

"Getting screened for colorectal cancer was a no-brainer. It was easy. The difficult part was the prep, and that wasn't even that bad. Honestly, it was a piece of cake: go in, go to sleep, and then go home. I plan to get screened again when it's time and encourage people in my life to do the same."

—Bill Lind, Oregon resident

CONTACT

Oregon Comprehensive Cancer Control Program

■ 800 Northeast Oregon Street
Suite 730
Portland, OR 97232

■ 971- 673-1121

■ http://public.health.oregon.gov/
DiseasesConditions/ChronicDisease/
Cancer/Pages/index.aspx

The pilot study confirmed earlier findings that an effective method of increasing CRC screening rates is to have people who have been screened talk about their experience with their peers and encourage them to get screened as well.

The media campaign included the two hospitals in Clatsop County; large employers; local institutions; associations such as the Chamber of Commerce, Rotary Club, and Kiwanis Club; insurance providers; county school districts; the Clatsop County Housing Authority; and the community college. Overall, 22 local organizations distributed materials to more than 24,000 local residents.

In a post-pilot telephone survey, 91 of 196 people recalled seeing or hearing campaign ads, news stories, and materials. People who had been screened were more likely to recall the campaign, which is a key finding given that the primary audience is Oregonians who have been screened.

Nearly 80% of respondents who recalled the campaign said they agreed or strongly agreed that the campaign made them more likely to recommend CRC screening. During the 3-month pilot period, Dr. Truman Sasaki, the campaign's provider champion, performed 71 more colonoscopies than during the same period the year before, totaling 220 colonoscopies, including 20 who requested screening because of the campaign or because someone they knew encouraged them to get screened. Dr. Sasaki found and removed polyps—some pre-cancerous—from nearly half of the patients, possibly preventing cancer and needless death. Dr. Sasaki found cancer in one patient, enabling the patient to begin treatment immediately.

Local businesses, media, clubs, and other institutions proved willing to give resources and attention to this important topic at reduced or no cost. As a consequence, the resiliency, well-being, and vibrancy of the community were strengthened.

"When my grandmother died of colorectal cancer back when I was a child, there wasn't really the option to get screened and prevent the cancer altogether. So, now that we have that option, why wouldn't everyone get screened? Some friends and coworkers tell me they're nervous. I was too. But, I say with all confidence that it's really not that bad."

— Gretchen Darnell, Oregon resident

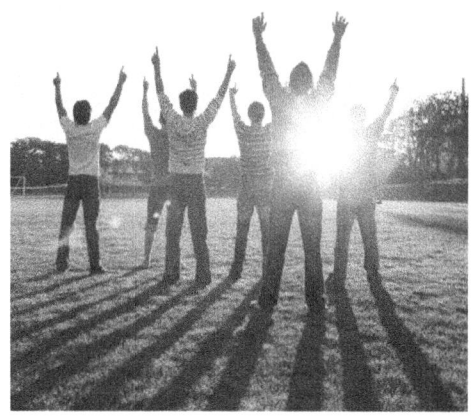

DEMONSTRATE OUTCOMES THROUGH EVALUATION

CDC plans to conduct research and surveillance activities that will develop and evaluate comprehensive approaches to cancer prevention and control. Results will guide interventions designed to address cross-cutting issues (such as health disparities and survivorship) at state, tribal, and territorial levels. Learn how two programs improved public health through evaluation. Find out more at http://www.cdc.gov/cancer/ncccp/about.htm.

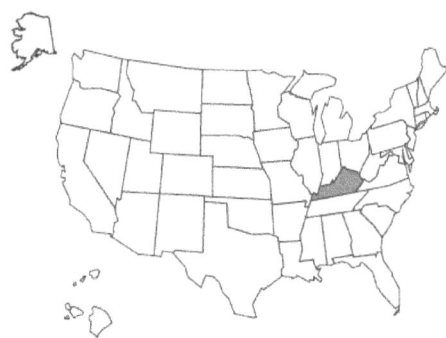

KENTUCKY

Collaboration in Evaluation: Using Partnerships

Kentucky has consistently had one of the highest rates of smoking among adults, now ranking 49th in the nation. So, it is not surprising that lung cancer kills more Kentuckians than any other type of cancer. Kentucky's lung cancer death rate is the highest in the nation.* Despite intense public educational campaigns and other efforts, tobacco use remains high: 26.8% of adults in Kentucky use tobacco, compared to the national average of 19.3%.[†]

Health care leaders expected that demand for smoking cessation options would increase as local communities enacted smoke-free ordinances, so the Kentucky Cancer Program (KCP) was asked to evaluate statewide smoking cessation programs. Although the Kentucky Department for Public Health provides information on a range of smoking cessation options, KCP was specifically asked to evaluate the Cooper/Clayton Method to Stop Smoking (CC Method) (http://www.stopsmoking4ever.org), since it combines use of nicotine replacement products with group cessation counseling, the combination that has been most effective. Many organizations in the state have used the CC Method with significant anecdotal success, but the program has not been evaluated formally in several years.

Since a large, statewide program was being evaluated, KCP asked the Kentucky Cancer Consortium, a diverse group of partners in cancer control, to coordinate their agendas and goals, and to collect and analyze data. The consortium, including the KCP, the University of Kentucky's College of Public Health, local health departments, and the Kentucky Department for Public Health's Tobacco Prevention and Cessation Program, determined that the program evaluation should consist of two parts: a retrospective study that would collect data from 2009–2010 to establish a baseline success rate, and a prospective study that would provide both the current success rate

> *The risk of developing lung cancer is about 23 times higher among men who smoke cigarettes and about 13 times higher among women who smoke cigarettes compared with never smokers.*

CONTACT

Kentucky Cancer Consortium

■ 2365 Harrodsburg Road
Suite B100
Lexington, KY 40504-3381

■ 859-219-0772 ext. 252

■ http://www.kycancerc.org

---

*U.S. Cancer Statistics Working Group. *United States Cancer Statistics: 1999–2008 Incidence and Mortality Web-based Report.* Atlanta: U.S. Department of Health and Human Services, Centers for Disease Control and Prevention and National Cancer Institute; 2012. Available at http://www.cdc.gov/uscs.

[†]Centers for Disease Control and Prevention. Vital Signs: Current cigarette smoking among adults aged ≥18 years—United States, 2005–2010. *Morbidity and Mortality Weekly Report.* 2011;60(35);1207–1212.

and smoking rates during a follow-up period to determine whether program participants stayed smoke-free. The retrospective study was started in the spring of 2011, and the prospective study started in January 2012.

The consortium developed an online evaluation tool, and people who took the CC Method classes were invited to enter information. Class facilitators could enter overall class information. Seventy-one class facilitators entered information about 231 classes taught in 2009–2010. Of 2,072 people who enrolled, 918 completed the class as nonsmokers, yielding a success rate of 44.31%. Those participants most likely to be helped by the program were women aged 45 to 64 years, and those who had smoked for 16 to 25 years.

CC Method to Stop Smoking Participants					
Gender	Men: 330 (36%)			Women 588 (64%)	
Age	≤24 years: 48 (5%)	25–44 years: 276 (30%)	45–64 years: 478 (52%)	≥65 years: 91 (10%)	Missing data: 25 (3%)
Smoking history	≤5 years: 30 (3%)	6–15 years: 157 (17%)	16–25 years: 295 (32%)	26–35 years: 245 (27%)	≥35 years: 188 (21%)	Missing data: 3 (0.33%)

This program evaluation could not have been done without the help of all partners. Using information from this evaluation about the CC Method's effectiveness, smokers will be better able to decide whether it is the right way for them to quit.

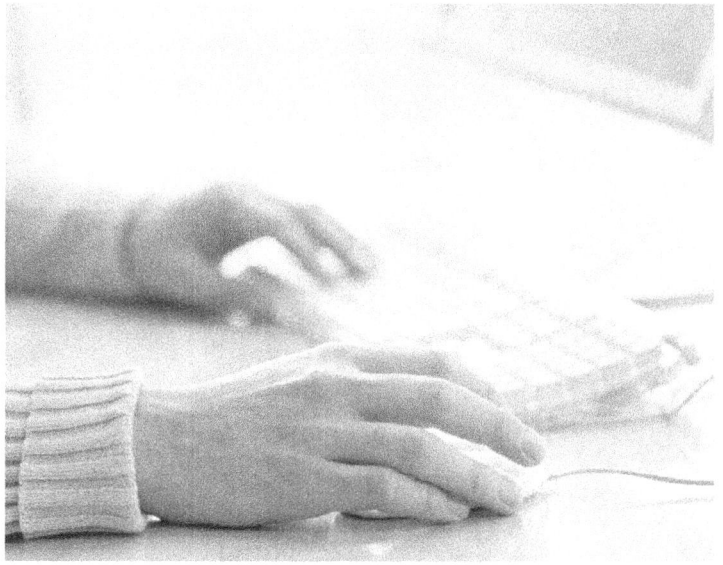

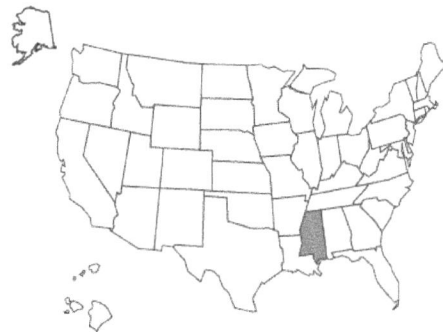

MISSISSIPPI

Seniors Tackling Cancer

Today we talk more often of "cancer survivors" than "cancer victims." Much progress has been made in cancer prevention and early detection, and better treatment and care for those affected by the disease. Nonetheless, more than 13,000 Mississippians are likely to be diagnosed with cancer in 2012. Though we rank 25th of states in cancer incidence, our cancer death rate, at third, is among the highest in the nation.

Winston County, Mississippi, having the fourth-highest cancer death rate in the state, is committed to finding local solutions to help fight cancer.

The Mississippi State University Extension Service developed the Seniors Tackling Cancer project to help communities find ways to prevent or detect cancer early, and improve survivors' quality of life. The effort is supported by the Mississippi State Department of Health's Comprehensive Cancer Control Program with funding from the Centers for Disease Control and Prevention.

As part of this effort, forums were held to involve the community in identifying current resources and challenges in fighting cancer. The forums used guided questions to help county residents better understand 1) what is currently working in the community, 2) what people would like to see happen, 3) what they are willing to do, 4) what ideas they may have, 5) what they see as obstacles and, 6) what they are going to do.

The forums were conducted using a modified World Café* format, in which a facilitator uses the guided questions to start discussions between six to eight people sitting at a table. Their thoughts were joined with those of people at neighboring tables to build a voice for the room. A diverse group of 32 people attended the forums.

---

*The World Café. World Café Method. Available at http://www.theworldcafe.com/method.html.

CONTACT

Mississippi State Department of Health Comprehensive Cancer Control Program

■ 570 East Woodrow Wilson Drive
PO Box 1700
Jackson, MS 39215-1700

■ 601-576-7781

■ http://www.msdh.state.ms.us/msdhsite/_static/43,0,292.html

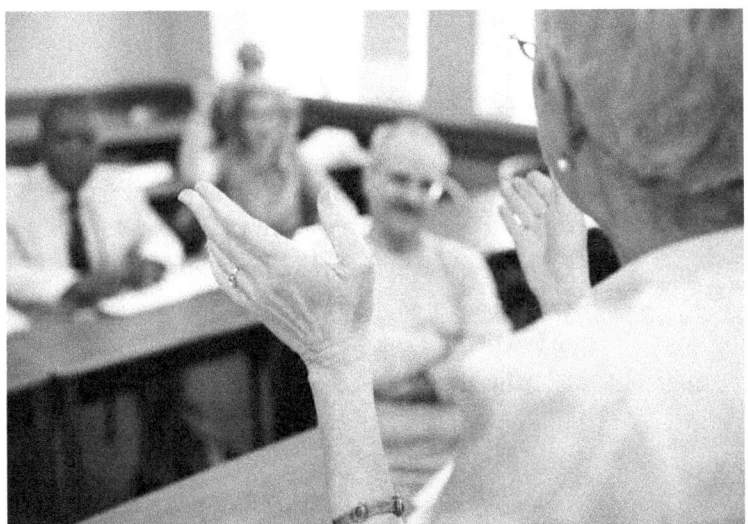

Most participants were aged ≥50 years, and many were cancer survivors or caretakers. Participants developed a "wish list" of what they would like to see happen in Winston County. Based on this list, three community action groups formed to develop local solutions to reduce cancer's impact on local residents. The groups have

- Developed a volunteer program to call and visit cancer patients and their caregivers and to give food to those with low incomes.

- Produced a directory of available support services in partnership with another community organization.

- Found ways to make wellness activities more social and increase local participation by advertising wellness-oriented community activities. To kick off this effort, the local newspaper published an article featuring the Seniors Tackling Cancer group's goals.

In the long term, the success of this project will be measured by the impact of the work of these groups in helping cancer patients and their families, improving their quality of life, and increasing opportunities for and participation in health-improving activities.

Of the 11.7 million people living with cancer in 2007, the largest groups of cancer survivors were:

- *Breast cancer survivors (22%).*

- *Prostate cancer survivors (19%).*

- *Colorectal cancer survivors (10%).*

RESOURCES
Resources for Creating Effective Success Stories

Simply Put

Developed by the Centers for Disease Control and Prevention, Office of the Associate Director for Communication. A guide to creating easy-to-understand materials.

http://www.cdc.gov/healthliteracy/pdf/Simply_Put.pdf

Impact and Value: Telling Your Program's Story

Developed by the Centers for Disease Control and Prevention, Division of Oral Health, this is a resource for program managers to create success stories that highlight their program's achievements. Although its examples are from state workers in oral health promotion, the methods for collecting and writing success stories can be applied to any public health program.

http://www.cdc.gov/Oralhealth/publications/library/pdf/success_story_workbook.pdf

How to Develop a Success Story

Developed by the Centers for Disease Control and Prevention, Division of Adolescent and School Health, to offer guidance on how to write a compelling success story.

http://www.cdc.gov/HealthyYouth/stories/pdf/howto_create_success_story.pdf

Evaluation Tutorials

The tutorials build skills around describing, planning, evaluating, and improving programs and contain interactive exercises, review pages, and downloadable resources and examples.

http://www.cdc.gov/HealthyYouth/evaluation/resources.htm#5

Plain Language: Improving Communication from the Federal Government to the Public

A Web site to help federal agencies write in plain language. Writing tips, examples, and resource lists guide writers to create effective documents, letters, and manuals that are accessible to all readers.

http://www.plainlanguage.gov

National Association of Chronic Disease Directors State Success Stories

The Web site provides selected stories from state chronic disease directors. This Web site lists reasons and uses for writing compelling success stories and provides clear examples of success stories in public health.

http://www.chronicdisease.org/?page=SuccessStories

WISEWOMAN Works: A Collection of Success Stories From Program Inception Through 2002

(Published in 2003. Note: some contact information may be out of date.)

http://www.cdc.gov/wisewoman/docs/success_stories.pdf

WISEWOMAN Works: A Collection of Success Stories on Empowering Women to Stop Smoking

(Published in 2005. Note: some contact information may be out of date.)

http://www.cdc.gov/wisewoman/docs/success_stories_vol2.pdf

PROGRAM WEB SITES

Alabama
http://www.adph.org

Alaska Native Tribal Health Consortium
http://www.anthctoday.org

Arizona
http://www.azdhs.gov/azcancercontrol

Arkansas
http://www.healthyarkansas.com

California
http://www.cdph.ca.gov/programs/csrb/
Pages/default.aspx

Cherokee Nation
http://cancer.cherokee.org

Hawaii
http://hawaii.gov/health/family-child-health/chronic-
disease/cccp/index.html

Indiana
http://www.indianacancer.org

Kentucky
http://www.kycancerc.org

Maryland
http://www.msa.md.gov/msa/mdmanual/26excom/
html/05can.html

Michigan
http://www.michigan.gov/mdch/0,1607,7-132-
2940_2955_2975-13561--,00.html

Minnesota
http://www.health.state.mn.us/divs/hpcd/compcancer

Mississippi
http://www.msdh.state.ms.us/msdhsite/_static/43,0,292.
html

Montana
http://www.dphhs.mt.gov/publichealth/cancer

Oregon
http://public.health.oregon.gov/DiseasesConditions/
ChronicDisease/Cancer/Pages/index.aspx

Tennessee
http://health.state.tn.us/CCCP

Utah
http://health.utah.gov/ucan